THE WONDERS OF HERBS

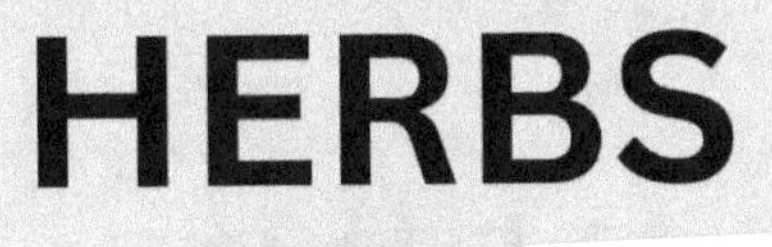

A Handbook of Herbs and Herbal Remedies

Leslie W. Kings

THE WONDERS OF

HERBS

A Handbook of Herbs and Herbal Remedies

Leslie W. Kings

TABLE OF CONTENTS

HERBALISM: AN INTRODUCTION

Herbalism refers to folk and traditional medicine based on the use of plants and plant extracts. Other names for herbalism are phytotherapy, botanical medicine, herbology, and phytomedicine. It entails the use of medicinal plants, which are the basis of traditional medicine. It is categorized as a type of alternative or complementary medicine. Nearly all non-industrialized societies employ herbal medicine to treat illness. People with chronic illnesses like cancer, asthma, diabetes, and end-stage kidney disease are more likely to take herbal medicines. In actuality, many pharmaceutical drugs are man-made derivatives of naturally occurring plant compounds. For instance, the foxglove plant served as the source for the cardiac medication digitalis. Opium, aspirin, digitalis, and quinine are just a few of the medications that are currently available to Western doctors or physicians and have a long history of use as herbal remedies. It has also been demonstrated that a number of factors, including age, gender, ethnicity, education, and socio-economic class, are related to how frequently people utilize herbal treatments.

As by-products of their typical metabolic processes, all plants synthesize chemical compounds. These chemical compounds can be divided into two groups: primary metabolites, which are present in all plants and include carbohydrates, proteins, and lipids, and secondary metabolites, which are present in a narrower variety of plants, some of which are unique to a single genus or species. Secondary metabolites have a variety of biological roles, such as acting as toxins or poisons to ward off predators or as pheromones in attracting insects for pollination. These secondary metabolites can be processed to create drugs and have therapeutic effects on people. Quinine from cinchona, inulin from dahlia roots, morphine and codeine from poppies, and digoxin from foxglove are a few examples. Many of the herbs and spices that people use in seasoning food also contain beneficial therapeutic compounds.

Several herbal medicines have been used in providing remedies to body-related issues. There are potential advantages to using black cohosh and other phytoestrogen-containing herbs to alleviate menopausal symptoms. Garlic has been shown to have antimicrobial characteristics, lower blood pressure mildly, prevent platelet aggregation, and lower total cholesterol levels. In preliminary investigations, artichoke and a number of other plants have been linked to lower total serum cholesterol levels. Echinacea extracts, in certain clinical trials, have been demonstrated to shorten the duration of colds, however, other investigations have found no benefit.

As beneficial as herbs are, some herbs can also be very dangerous. It is a popular misconception that using natural products and practicing herbalism, in general, is safe. Nature or natural products, however, do not always guarantee safety. Nature is not a totally harmless place, and many plants have chemical defence mechanisms against predators that may be harmful to people. Hemlock and nightshade are two examples that can be fatal to people. Herbs, much like pharmaceuticals, can cause negative side effects in uncontrolled dosage and poor quality.

Few generalizations can be made about herbalism because it is such a diverse field. However, a general agreement can be deduced. The majority of herbalists acknowledge that when time is of essence, pharmaceuticals or Western medicine are more efficient. An illustration would be if a patient, has dangerously high blood pressure.

They assert, however, that over the long term, herbs can aid in a patient's ability to fend off sickness, and also offer nutritional and immunological support that medications are unable to. They see prevention and cure as realistic and achievable goals with the application of herbalism.

Herbalists typically use extracts from plant parts like the roots or leaves rather than isolating specific phytochemicals. Pharmaceutical medicine favours single substance since it is simpler to quantify dosage. Herbalists, on the other hand, disagree with the idea of a single active component. They contend that the various phytochemicals that are found in many herbs will interact to boost the herb's medicinal effects and lessen its toxicity. Herbalists hold that if an active ingredient is utilized separately from the rest of the plant, it may lose its effectiveness or become less safe. For instance, the plant meadowsweet contains salicylic acid, which is used to manufacture aspirin. Aspirin can make the stomach lining bleed; however, meadowsweet naturally includes other substances that shield the body from the irritating effect of salicylic acid. Practitioners of herbal medicine argue that the complete plant has a bigger impact than the sum of its parts

Herbalists contest the idea that synthetic chemicals may replicate the synergism of medicinal plants. They contend that phytochemical interactions and trace components may change the way medicines react in ways that are now impossible to duplicate with a small number of putative active ingredients. Pharmaceutical researchers acknowledge the idea of drug synergism but point out that, assuming the composition or formulation of a particular herbal preparation is consistent, clinical studies may be utilized to examine its efficacy.

FORMS OF HERBS ADMINISTERING

The extraction technique has an impact on the precise composition of an herbal product. Water is a polar solvent; hence a tisane will be abundant in polar components. On the other hand, oil is a non-polar solvent that may take up non-polar substances. Alcohol falls in the middle. The extraction solvent, temperature, and duration of the extraction process vary for different plant and herb extracts. The components of a herbal extract or product may differ greatly across batches and producers because there is no standardization in place.

Herbs can be administered in a wide variety of forms, including:

1. **Tisanes:** This is also known as herbal tea or herbal infusion. This is a hot-water extract of herbs such as chamomile, mint, and green and black tea. The extracts are usually the leaves, flowers, and stems of herbal plants.

2. **<u>Decoctions:</u>** This is made from the long-term boiling of plant extracts, usually roots and bark. Both decoction and tisane or infusion are hot-water extracts of herbs.

3. **<u>Tinctures:</u>** These are alcoholic extracts of herbs like Echinacea. They are often produced by mixing the herb with 100% pure ethanol or diluted ethanol solvent. A finished tincture contains at least 40-60% (and occasionally up to 90%) ethanol. The potency of many medicinal herbs usually lasts longer and is stronger in alcohol extracts than in water extracts.

4. **<u>Herbal Wine and Elixirs:</u>** These are alcoholic extracts of herbs, often containing 12-38% ethanol. It is known as herbal wine when wine is used as the alcoholic solvent, and elixir when spirits (vodka, gin, etc.) are used as the alcoholic solvent.

5. **<u>Macerates:</u>** These are cold infusions of herbs with high mucilage content (e.g. sage, thyme, etc.). In cold water, chopped plants are introduced. They are then allowed to stand for seven to twelve hours (depending on the herb used). On average, 10 hours are used for macerates.

6. **Topicals:** Herbal medicines can also be administered directly on the skin in form of topicals.

- **Essential Oils:** This is the application of essential oil extracts diluted in a carrier oil. Essential oils in their concentrated form can burn the skin or are simply high doses to be used directly. Diluting in olive oil or another food-grade oil can allow these essential oils to be used safely as a topical.

- **Balms, Creams, Lotions, Oils, and Salves:** The majority of topical applications use herbal oils. Some phytochemicals can be extracted into oil by soaking herbs in food-grade oil for a few weeks to many months. The oil can then be used topically or in the production of salves, creams, lotions, massage oils, antibacterial salves, and wound-healing compounds.

- **Poultices and Compresses:** Whole herbs (or relevant parts of the plant) can also be used to form poultices or compresses. They are often crushed or dried, rehydrated with a little quantity of water, or fat, like vegetable oil, and then applied externally to damaged skin areas for treatment. Application can be directly to a bandage, cloth, or on the skin. They are the herbal medicines with the shortest shelf-life. The application of poultices and compresses is the same, but typically a decoction or infusion is used in conjunction with a compress.

7. **<u>Whole-Herbs Consumption:</u>** Herbs can be consumed in either fresh form (juice, fresh leaves, and other plant parts) or dry form (herbal powder, etc.). Besides their initial application as medicinal herbs, it has become evident that eating vegetables easily fits within the category of obtaining health through consumables. Vitamins, minerals, and antioxidants that we obtain from food are phytochemicals. Although different herbs play different roles, it is obvious that some whole herbs we consume have greater potency than others. Alfalfa is regarded as a nutritious food. Garlic reduces cholesterol, enhances blood circulation, and combats yeast, bacteria, and viruses. Shitake mushrooms are fantastic in soups and other food preparations for the cold and flu season since they enhance the immune system and taste delicious.

8. **<u>Sirups:</u>** These are herbal extracts made from honey or syrup. Sugar is mixed with a water & herb mixture in a 65% to 35% ratio

respectively. The entire mixture is boiled afterward and then macerated for three weeks.

9. **Extracts:** Liquid, dry, and nebulized extracts are all types of extracts. Liquid extracts are similar to tinctures, but they have lower ethanol content. Dry extracts are plant-based extracts that have been evaporated into a dry form. Then they can be transformed or packaged into a tablet or capsule. Nebulisates are dry extracts made from freeze-drying.

10. **Herbal Juice:** Simply juicing plants or herbs yields fresh juice. This is an excellent way to obtain vitamins and minerals from the plant, but the juice must be consumed shortly after extraction because fermentation and oxidation cause the vitamin content to fast degrade.

11. **Inhalation or Aromatherapy:** This does not involve direct inhalation of herbs, rather steam created from the process of boiling the herbs is inhaled. Inhalation can be used to alleviate depression, heal a cough or sinus infection, or deep-cleanse the skin. Essential oils can also be used in aromatherapy.

12. **Herbal Baths:** These are another option to use herbs to treat a greater area of the body. Application includes the utilization of oatmeal or Aveeno in a baby bath or lavender or camomile flowers for a relaxing bath.

HEALTH CONCERNS OF HERBAL MEDICINE

The idea that using natural products and herbs in general entails safety is a frequent fallacy. Some herbs should be used with the same level of caution as pharmaceutical drugs because they contain potent ingredients. Many herbs and plant products have in their components toxic substances that can seriously harm both humans and animals. Given that they do include powerful chemicals, herbs are just like pharmaceutical drugs in that they may cause undesired side effects such as rashes and allergic reactions, diarrhoea, sleeplessness, muscle and joint pain, asthma, headache, nausea, and vomiting. Lack of control over dosage and purity makes these issues worse, especially when taken without the correct guidance of a herbalist or naturopath or when the herbs are not standardized. Some herbal medicines may be difficult to correctly dose. The growth circumstances, age, and processing of the plant are only a few of the many factors that might impact the quality of herbal medicines. As a result, there is no established method for giving the appropriate dosage. If someone is contemplating taking herbal medicine, self-prescription should be avoided. They should rather consult a herbalist first.

Additionally, there is a risk of summation when drugs and herbs with similar effects are administered together, and it can result in an overdose. For example, combining a blood pressure-lowering herbal treatment with a prescription drug that has the same effect can lead to dangerously low blood pressure. The positive and negative effects of prescription and over-the-counter drugs can be increased or decreased by taking herbal supplements, the National Center for Complementary and Integrative Health cautions. An instance is St. John's Wort which mostly lessens other medications' effectiveness but enhances the effects of antidepressants. Another instance is the Ginkgo biloba which should be used with caution by persons who take blood-thinning drugs (such as aspirin and warfarin). This is due to a higher risk of bleeding. A naturopath would be very useful in this situation because of his knowledge about the proper herbs to use, dosages, and timing, as well as any potential interactions between the herbs and other medications. In general, naturopathic doctors will prescribe particular single herbs or combinations of herbs to be taken in the various forms explained earlier and may be administered in conjunction with other natural treatments.

The majority of naturopaths employ plant parts like the roots and leaves rather than isolating specific phytochemicals since the synergy of the combined compounds increases the effectiveness of the phytochemicals and reduces toxicity if any. An example is vitamin C which, when gotten from a dietary source like pepper or orange, is more complete and balanced for the body than the vitamin C supplement form which is generally an isolated compound in a pill form.

The National Health Service (NHS) of the United Kingdom indicates that a person may not be able to take herbal medicine if they are pregnant, nursing, using other prescription or over-the-counter drugs, under 18, over 65, or undergoing surgery. The NHS also advises anyone taking herbal medications to inform their doctor before undergoing surgery. This is due to the possibility that some herbal remedies could alter blood pressure and blood coagulation both before and after surgery by interfering with anaesthetic medications.

Additionally, since herbal medicine is not subject to the same Food and Drug Administration (FDA) regulation as prescription and over-the-counter drugs, it is crucial to use caution when using it. This implies that there is a vast range in the effectiveness, safety, and quality of herbal products.

HEALTH BENEFITS OF HERBS

For thousands of years, people have utilized herbs as food flavours, medicine, and preservatives. Herbaceous plants known as culinary herbs are used to flavour and decorate a variety of dishes. In addition to flavour and colour, each herb tends to have its own therapeutic properties. The term "Herbs" has been defined differently with regard to medicine and culinary studies. In culinary use, herbs typically refer to the leafy green or flowering parts of a plant (either fresh or dried), while spices are typically dried and made from other plant parts, such as seeds, roots, bark, and fruits.

Herbs are of benefits in the management and prevention of diabetes, cancer, and heart disease. They are anti-inflammatory and anti-tumour properties, and may also reduce blood clots. Although research is ongoing, studies have revealed that:

- Garlic, linseed, lemongrass, and fenugreek may aid in lowering cholesterol levels.

- Fenugreek, flaxseed, linseed, and cinnamon can help regulate insulin activity and blood sugar levels.

- Rosmarinic acid, the active ingredient in Rosemary, aids in the prevention of allergies and nasal congestion.

- Garlic is helpful in lowering blood pressure, for immunity, and for improving heart health.

- Numerous herbs, including mint, basil, sage, oregano, garlic, leeks, onions, and chives can help prevent cancer.

- Sage extract can enhance mental and cognitive abilities, particularly in people with Alzheimer's disease.

- Herbs, particularly cloves, cinnamon, sage, thyme, and oregano are abundant in antioxidants and can lower low-density lipoproteins (often known as bad cholesterol)

- Ginger has anti-inflammatory and anti-inflammatory properties, relieves pain, and can be used to treat nausea and other gastrointestinal tract problems.

- Curcumin, found in turmeric, is a strong antioxidant and has powerful anti-inflammatory effects.

- Individuals suffering from Irritable Bowel Syndrome (IBS) can get pain relief from peppermint's natural oil. When used in aromatherapy, it also has effective anti-nausea properties.

- Capsaicin, the active ingredient in Cayenne pepper, suppresses hunger and speeds up fat burning. It has also demonstrated anti-cancerous properties.

- Holy basil boosts immunity and inhibits antibacterial and antifungal growth.

- Cumin helps in cholesterol, stress, and diabetes management.

Fresh herbs have higher antioxidant levels compared to dried or processed herbs.

MODE OF ACTION OF HERBS

The fact that plants cannot defend themselves or deploy active weaponry when confronted by herbivores, whether it be insects, molluscs, worms, or vertebrates, is a simple but nonetheless significant finding. Vertebrates and humans have highly effective innate and acquired immune systems that may rely on when threatened by microbes; plants do not have such an immune system. However, despite being threatened by herbivores and microbes, plants have presumably endured on this planet for thousands of years. In order for plants to defend themselves against herbivores as well as against bacteria, fungi, and viruses, thousands of structurally different secondary metabolites are believed to have evolved during plant growth.

Plants manufacture secondary metabolites in a variety of forms. Secondary metabolites act both as signalling molecules (to attract pollination and seed-dispersing animals) and as defensive mechanisms against herbivores, other plants, and bacteria. Some secondary metabolites also act as antioxidants and UV protectants. A wide range of biological and pharmacological features are often displayed by secondary metabolites. As a result, certain plants or products derived from them have been and are currently utilized as herbs to treat illnesses, infections, and other conditions.

Many plants have a reputation for being poisonous or having hallucinogenic effects. These plants frequently have certain alkaloids, terpenoids, or other secondary metabolites that specifically modulate a corresponding molecular target in humans or animals. Neuroreceptors, enzymes that break down neurotransmitters, ion channels, ion pumps, or components of the cytoskeleton (primarily tubulin or microtubules) are frequently the targets. Many of these secondary metabolites are currently isolated from plants and employed as chemical substances in modern medicine with well-established applications. Different secondary metabolites have different specified targets.

Secondary metabolites in herbs that support their contemporary and conventional usage include:

1. **<u>Coumarin:</u>** Numerous plants, such as lavender, horse chestnut, dandelion, solanaceous plants, poppies, sweet clover, parsley, and angelica contain coumarins. Warfarin is made from its fermentation product dicoumarol, a strong anti-clotting agent. Coumarins have spasmolytic, antibacterial, vasodilative, and anti-edema properties. They are used as venous and lymphatic vessel tonics in medicine.

2. **<u>Alkaloids:</u>** They are usually bitter tasting and are generated from amino acids. A combination of alkaloids with tannins will cause the precipitation of the alkaloids. Therefore, tannins can be used to treat acute alkaloid toxicity. Some subgroups such as pyrrolizidine alkaloids have harmful and toxic potentials while some others like isoquinoline alkaloids (berberine, hydrastine, and sanguinarine) are medicinal and are found in herbs including barberry, goldenseal, Oregon Grape root, and bloodroot. These alkaloids have antioxidant, anti-inflammatory, antimicrobial, ionotropic, and antineoplastic effects, among other effects.

3. **<u>Saponins:</u>** They typically taste sweet and form lather in water. They can be found in herbs like ivy, licorice, astragalus, Panax

ginseng, and wild yam. They frequently contain steroidal compounds that can regulate the effects on steroidal receptors. They have shown antiviral and anti-inflammatory effects. They function as expectorants, promote the production of mucus in the lungs, and lower cholesterol. Toxicity of saponin glycosides can result in haemolysis, however, they are extremely safe when taken at the right dosage.

4. **Flavonoids:** They are found in many plants, but hawthorn, elderflower, bilberry, and grapes have the highest concentrations. Flavonoids and proanthocyanidins (which are oligomers of flavonoids) are mainly antioxidants. They may also have anti-inflammatory, antineoplastic, and anti-allergic effects., and they also reduce capillary permeability and fragility.

5. **Anthraquinones:** Aloe vera, yellow dock, cascara, senna, and turkey rhubarb are just a few of the well-known laxative herbs that contain anthraquinones, which are red or yellow pigments. Pharmacological studies have confirmed their laxative properties, and they are also anti-inflammatory.

6. **Tannins:** They have astringent properties because of their capacity to bind molecules like proteins. Numerous herbs contain them, such as black tea, oak bark, witch hazel, oak galls, and blackberry. They are effective in the treatment of diarrhoea due to their gastrointestinal tract anti-inflammatory and anti-ulcer properties. Their styptic activity enables them to be used as astringents for wounds.

7. **Volatile Oil:** Aromatic herbs, including common kitchen herbs like lemon balm, fennel, peppermint, rosemary, cinnamon, and cardamom, contain volatile oils. They are used as carminatives to promote digestion and lessen flatulence and have proven to have spasmolytic effects on the smooth muscles of the trachea and gastrointestinal tract, expectorant effects on mucociliary clearance, and anti-inflammatory and antiseptic effects.

8. **Sterols and Sterolin:** All plants, fruits, and vegetables contain sterols and sterolins, which are chemically alike to cholesterol. They are also known as phytosterols. The primary phytosterol in higher plants is beta-sitosterol. Phytosterols have been shown

through animal research to have anti-inflammatory, anti-cancer, antipyretic, glucose-lowering, and immune-modulating properties.

GINGER

Ginger (Zingiber officinale) is a flowering plant whose rhizome is utilized as herbs for traditional medicine and spices for culinary purposes. Ginger originated from Maritime South East Asia (Brunei, Indonesia, Malaysia, Singapore, East Timor, and the Philippines). Its use in Asian, Indian, and Arabic herbal traditions dates back a long time.

The natural oils in ginger, of which gingerol is the most significant, are what give it its distinct aroma and flavour. The primary bioactive ingredient in ginger is gingerol. It is responsible for ginger's therapeutic qualities. Other key constituents are shogaols and zingerones.

Research has shown that ginger has potent anti-inflammatory and antioxidant properties. For instance, it might assist in lowering oxidative stress or deterioration, which is brought on by the body having too many free radicals.

Forms of Ginger Administration

Ginger-containing herbs can be made using fresh or dried ginger root or from the steam distillation of the oil present in the root. Ginger is administered in the form of liquid extracts, tinctures, poultices, syrups, pills, oils, and herbal teas (tisanes). Ginger has often been taken orally, but it also has topical applications in the form of topical gels, ointments, and essential oils for aromatherapy. Additionally, since ginger is also a spice, it can be consumed from foods and beverages.

Mode of Action of Ginger

Three key therapeutic substances found in ginger – gingerols, shogaols, and zingerones – are all closely related terpenoids with strong anti-inflammatory effects. The bioactive component of ginger root (rhizome) that gives it its anti-emetic, anti-inflammatory, and antispasmodic actions is called gingerol, a group of structurally similar polyphenolic compounds identified from ginger. Although further research is required to fully understand ginger's mechanism of action, some evidence points to the fact that it may help Irritable

Bowel Syndrome (IBS) sufferers by lowering pain and regulating gastrointestinal motility.

Depending on whether ginger is cooked or dried during processing, gingerols split into two distinct components. The gingerols change into shogaol molecules when ginger is dried, but they become zingerones when ginger is cooked. The flavour and medicinal value of ginger are substantially impacted by these processes. Shogaols have a more pungent flavour than zingerones, which makes dried ginger seem less appealing. The therapeutic efficacy of dried ginger is higher because shogaols have a minor advantage over zingerones in terms of potency. The flavour of zingerones is sweeter. Capsaicin, caffeic acid, curcumin, beta-carotene, and vitamin C are among the additional ingredients and nutrients found in ginger.

Main Effects and Uses of Ginger

1. Ginger has been used in China, for instance, to alleviate nausea, diarrhoea, and stomach discomforts as well as to aid with digestion.

2. Ginger has been used to treat heart ailments, arthritis, colic, and diarrhoea.

3. It has been used to alleviate the symptoms of the common cold, the flu, headaches, and painful menstrual cycles.

4. Ginger has anti-inflammatory, anti-diabetic, and blood thinning effects.

5. LDL (bad) cholesterol, total cholesterol, and blood triglyceride levels can all be markedly lowered by ginger.

6. The gingerol in ginger has anti-cancer effect and can help reduce the risk of infection.

7. Ginger helps shield the brain against deterioration brought on by aging. Additionally, it may enhance cognitive function.

8. Ginger also possesses antispasmodic and analgesic properties.

Side Effects of Ginger

The FDA views ginger as safe when used in moderation, but it does not support or regulate its use as a medicine or dietary supplement. Ginger rarely causes negative side effects. It might induce minor heartburn, diarrhoea, and oral irritation at high doses. By taking ginger with meals or as a supplement, you may be able to avoid some of the moderate gastrointestinal side effects including belching, heartburn, or stomach discomfort.

Ginger should not be administered to children under the age of 2 years. Pregnant or breastfeeding women, individuals with heart conditions or gallstones, and those with diabetes should consult a doctor before using ginger. If you have a bleeding disorder or are taking aspirin, clopidogrel, warfarin, phenprocoumon, nifedipine, or other blood-thinning medications, DON'T consume ginger.

Ginger has blood sugar and pressure-lowering effects and may interact with prescriptions and over-the-counter drugs such as losartan, cyclosporine, metronidazole, diabetes medications, and high blood pressure medications.

GARLIC

Garlic (Allium sativum) is a type of herb that is closely related to leeks, onions, shallots, and chives. It is native to South Asia, North-eastern Iran, and Central Asia. It has a long history of use as both herbs and spices. Due to its ability to prevent cardiovascular diseases, control blood pressure, lower blood sugar and cholesterol levels, be effective against bacterial, fungal, viral, and parasitic infections, strengthen the immune system, and possess antitumor and antioxidant properties, garlic is thought to be a wonderful medicinal plant. The bulb of the garlic plant is the component of the plant that is utilized most frequently. The majority of garlic bulbs, except for those with single clove, are composed of several fleshy portions called cloves. Garlic cloves are consumed (raw or cooked) and also used medicinally.

Garlic is frequently prescribed for illnesses of the heart and blood. The active ingredient in garlic is allicin which is responsible for its odour, hot sensation, and therapeutic properties. Garlic may be aged to make some of its products odourless, however, this process can also alter the properties of garlic. Garlic's pungency is reduced by cooking because allicin is eliminated.

Many different cultures have employed garlic as traditional medicine, including Egypt, Greece, Rome, Japan, and China.

Forms of Garlic Administration

Garlic can be administered raw or in cooked form. The cloves are edible. It can also be utilized as pills and capsules after being dried or powdered. Oils and liquid extracts can also be made from raw garlic cloves. They can also be administered in the form of tinctures, poultices, and syrups.

Main Effects and Uses of Garlic

There are numerous possible health benefits of garlic.

1. Garlic may help lower the chance of developing certain cancers, such as stomach and colon cancer, according to some studies.

2. Garlic has blood pressure and cholesterol-lowering effect.

3. It also hardens the arteries. This is a precaution against atherosclerosis.

4. It may have antibiotic qualities that can be utilized to treat bacterial illnesses like the common cold. The ability of allicin to suppress RNA synthesis prevents the growth of bacteria and viruses.

5. It has antioxidant and anti-inflammatory effects which are essential in the treatment of osteoarthritis and other diseases.

6. Oral dosage of garlic may help tackle non-alcoholic fatty liver disease (NAFLD). NAFLD is the accumulation of fat in the liver in those who consume little to no alcohol.

7. It may help fight periodontitis, a severe gum infection.

8. Garlic has topical application in the treatment of fungal skin infections such as ringworm, athlete's foot, and jock itch). Ajoene, an ingredient in garlic, is responsible for this antifungal property.

Side Effects of Garlic

Although garlic is generally thought to be safe to eat, some people may have certain adverse effects. Orally consumed garlic is probably safe for the majority of people. With raw garlic, these negative effects are frequently harsher. The following are a few potential negative effects of garlic:

1. Heartburn, diarrhoea, and indigestion.

2. Bad breath and body odour.

3. Symptoms of an allergic reaction include skin rash, itching, and swelling in those who are sensitive to garlic.

4. Garlic has blood-thinning effects. This causes a reduction in the rate at which blood clot. People on blood-thinning medications (such as aspirin, coumadin, and warfarin) are advised to consult a doctor before including garlic in the diet or using it as an herb as it may raise the risk of bleeding.

5. Garlic may interact with prescriptions and over-the-counter drugs such as saquinavir (an HIV medication), atazanavir, tacrolimus, sofosbuvir, and isoniazid. It reduces the rate of absorption or breakdown of these drugs in the body.

6. Garlic has low blood pressure-lowering effects and may interact with prescriptions and over-the-counter medications that tackle high blood pressure (antihypertensive drugs). This may cause the blood pressure to go too low.

7. Garlic consumption along with diabetes medication may result in dangerously low blood sugar levels.

8. Irritable Bowel Syndrome (IBS) patients may experience gastrointestinal irritation as a result of garlic compounds usage.

TURMERIC

Turmeric (Curcuma longa) is a used in folk medicine as an herb and also as a spice. It has a golden yellow colour due to the presence of curcumin, its active ingredient. In India, where it was probably first employed as a dye, turmeric has been utilized for more than 2500 years. Over the years, other medical benefits of turmeric have gradually come to light. The rhizome is the part of the plant that is utilized as an herb or spice. Both Ayurvedic and Chinese medicine have traditionally utilized the anti-inflammatory property of turmeric to heal wounds, skin conditions, digestive and liver problems, and skin diseases.

Forms of Turmeric Administration

Turmeric is administered in form of tisanes and dried powder.

Main Effects and Uses of Turmeric

1. It has strong antioxidant and anti-inflammatory effects. These play a role in the prevention of diseases and health conditions such as

Alzheimer's disease, heart disease, cancer, and various degenerative conditions.

2. It is used to treat indigestion, flatulence, diarrhoea, and other gastrointestinal tract problems. A mixture of the rhizome (juice or powder form) and plain water or buttermilk is prepared.

3. Turmeric has blood cholesterol-lowering effect and also tackles hyperlipidemia – high lipid levels in the blood.

4. Due to its high iron content, turmeric is helpful in anaemia treatment. To treat this ailment, a teaspoon of fresh turmeric juice diluted with honey is administered daily.

5. It helps prevent the build-up of fats in the liver in people that take little or no alcohol (NAFLD).

6. Pain Relief: People with osteoarthritis may find that turmeric helps to lessen pain and stiffness.

7. Turmeric has been administered topically for ulcers and inflammation in Unani medicine, as well as internally for diseases like liver blockage and jaundice.

8. Eye sores can be treated with turmeric powder. 6g of the powder is boiled in about half a litre of water until the volume is reduced to

half. A few drops of this water is administered three or four times on the affected eyes to find comfort.

9. Applying turmeric powder on boils accelerates the recovery process. A few dry turmeric roots are roasted and the ashes are dissolved in a cup of water. The solution is applied to the area with boils. The boils can ripen and burst thanks to this treatment.

10. A remedy for dysentery has included roasted turmeric as one of its ingredients.

11. Treatment of skin conditions like ringworm and scabies can benefit from turmeric. In these situations, the affected areas are externally treated with fresh turmeric juice.

12. It has been utilized in dental paste or powder.

13. Turmeric is a helpful treatment for persistent cough and throat irritations thanks to its antiseptic properties. In this case, a mixture of 30ml of warm milk and half a teaspoon of fresh turmeric powder works wonders. To make this, milk is put into a hot ladle containing turmeric and boiled over a low flame. Smoke from burning turmeric can be inhaled in the event of a running nose. This causes more nasal discharge and provides relief more quickly.

When combined with caraway seeds or ajwain, turmeric is effective in treating colds in infants. For the treatment of such conditions, boiling water is mixed with a quarter teaspoon of ajwain and a teaspoon of turmeric powder. The mixture is allowed to cool and then sweetened with honey. 30ml of this hot-water extract is administered three times a day.

14. It has been demonstrated that it can both prevent prostate cancer and slow the spread of prostate cancer when mixed with cauliflower.

15. Measles can be treated with turmeric. The sun-dried turmeric roots are pounded into fine powder. This can be taken orally when combined with a few drops of honey and the juice of a few bitter gourd leaves.

16. Use turmeric paste blended with lime and salt to effectively cure sprains and the swelling brought on by sprains.

17. It increases bile synthesis in the liver and encourages bile discharge via the gallbladder. This enhances the body's capacity to metabolize fats.

Side Effects of Turmeric

Turmeric may interact with prescriptions and over-the-counter drugs such as anticoagulant and anti-diabetic medications, talinolol, sulfasalazine, tacrolimus, antitumor antibiotics, estrogen pills, amlodipine, tamoxifen, and hepatotoxic medications.

ALOE VERA

Aloe vera is thought to be indigenous only to the Al Hajar Mountains in north-eastern Oman and the south-east Arabian Peninsula. However, it has been widely farmed around the world and has naturalized in North Africa, the Canary Islands, the Madeira Islands, Cape Verde, as well as in Sudan and surrounding nations. In the 17th century, the plant was brought to China and several regions of southern Europe. Other places where it occurs naturally include desert and tropical areas of temperate continents.

Two major substances can be derived from Aloe vera – the clear gel and the yellow latex. Topical treatments for skin diseases such as burns, wounds, rashes, or dry skin are frequently made from aloe gel. Aloe latex is used either on its own or combined with additional ingredients to create a product that can be consumed to treat constipation. Aloe latex can be purchased as "aloe dry juice" or in a dried form known as resin. Commercially available yoghurts, beverages, and even desserts include aloe vera gel as part of their ingredients, but consuming aloe latex or whole-leaf extract can be harmful in high or sustained doses. Aloe vera topical use in moderation is probably safe.

Aloe vera can be made into a lotion, gel, soap, or cosmetic products for topical applications to the skin. People who are allergic to aloe vera may experience skin reactions such as contact dermatitis, symptoms of which are mild redness and itching, breathing difficulties, or swelling of the face, tongue, lips, or throat.

Forms of Aloe Vera Administration

Aloe vera can be administered orally (in the form of capsule or liquid) and topically. Oral dosage should be in moderation.

Main Effects and Uses of Aloe Vera

1. Wound healing effect: Its soothing, cooling, and moisturising qualities enable it to be used in healing wounds. For severe cuts and burns, aloe vera should never be used. Medical attention is needed instead.

2. Anti-inflammatory effects.

3. Moisturising and skin-hydrating effects: Aloe vera is frequently used to treat burns due to these qualities. The application of aloe

vera a few times daily to skin burn areas can aid treatment. Fresh aloe vera can be used to clear acne on the face.

4. Anti-aging effect.

5. Immune-modulating effect.

6. Aloe vera has antibacterial, antiviral, and antifungal properties.

7. Antioxidant property.

8. Blood-thinning or anti-clotting effect.

9. Antitumor effect.

10. Laxative effect and digestive health improvement: Consuming aloe vera may aid your digestive system, reduce stomach pain, and treat stomach conditions like constipation. Aloe vera can also prevent ulcers by inhibiting the growth of H. pylori, a gut bacteria.

11. It improves oral health: For better oral hygiene and dental plaque reduction, aloe vera toothpaste and mouthwash should be used. Aloe vera is a natural option compared to triclosan.

Side Effects and Precautions of Aloe Vera

Aloe vera use on the skin is typically not linked to any serious negative effects. It may be harmful when used orally as its laxative effect may cause diarrhoea and abdominal cramps, which might reduce drug absorption and effectiveness. Aloe products should not be consumed if you are taking prescription medications, including those for blood clots (e.g. warfarin), diabetes, heart disease, and potassium-lowering medications (like digoxin). Aloe vera shouldn't be used orally by women who are pregnant or nursing, or by children under the age of 12 years.

Those with tulips, garlic, or onions allergies are likely to be allergic to aloe vera also. Aloe vera should not be consumed two weeks before scheduled surgery because of its blood-thinning effect. This will slow down the rate at which blood will clot after the surgical treatment.

ALFALFA

Alfalfa (Medicago sativa) is also known as Lucerne. Medicago sativa has been utilized as a digestive aid in Traditional Chinese Medicine, a healthy tonic in American traditional medicine, and a culinary food in India. It is frequently consumed as a garnish in humans and appears to stop the stomach from absorbing cholesterol. Its seeds or dried leaves can be consumed as herbal supplements. The seeds can also be sprouted to make alfalfa sprouts. Alfalfa contains a significant amount of bioactive plant compounds, such as saponins, coumarins, flavonoids, phytosterols, and alkaloids.

Forms of Alfalfa Administration

There are various forms of preparing and administering alfalfa herbs. They include tinctures, herbal tea, dried herb, tablet, poultice, and powder forms.

Main Effects and Uses of Alfalfa

Alfalfa has a cholesterol-lowering effect. This is due to its high saponin concentration. Saponin promotes weight loss by assisting in the breakdown of lipids.

Due to its rich nutritional profile, alfalfa leaf is occasionally used to help healthy lactation in women.

It is a beneficial herb to use for balancing female hormones as it contains phytoestrogen.

Alfalfa has anti-inflammatory effects. It is a popular ingredient used in herbal arthritis treatments. It can reduce osteoarthritis-related pain and inflammation.

The body (liver, blood, and urinary tract) is cleansed, alkalized, and detoxified by alfalfa.

Side Effects of Alfalfa

Alfalfa sprouts are mostly healthy and harmless; however, some people may experience negative effects. Some persons, such as those who are pregnant, take blood thinners, have autoimmune diseases, or have weakened immune systems, may be adversely affected by alfalfa. It is not advised for long-term use or in large doses. L-canavanine, an amino acid found in alfalfa sprouts, has been shown to cause inflammation in persons with autoimmune diseases, mostly lupus. Consequently, alfalfa might cause acute lupus symptoms when consumed or taken as a supplement.

Alfalfa sprouts being contaminated by bacteria like salmonella or E. Coli is a cause for concern.

Alfalfa may interact with prescriptions and over-the-counter medications such as blood-thinning and blood cholesterol-lowering medications to reduce their rate of absorption and effectiveness.

AMARANTH

Amaranth grain contains phytochemicals such as polyphenols, tannins, saponins, and oxalates. Cooking reduces the amount of these chemicals and their antinutrient effect. Although every part of the plant is thought to be edible, some parts could have sharp spines that need to be removed before eating. Many regions of the world grow and eat various amaranth species as leafy vegetables.

Forms of Amaranth Administration

Amaranth is available for human use as food, essential oil, and powder.

It has mostly been used in both traditional and modern cultures as a food source for its leaves and seeds. However, nutritional and herbal products are increasingly using amaranth as an ingredient.

Main Effects and Uses of Amaranth

Squalene, a precursor to healthy cholesterol, is present in amaranth. Human studies have demonstrated the benefits of amaranth grain and oil for cardiovascular patients as well as its cholesterol-lowering effect.

It keeps the body regular by stimulating bowel movement. Fiber is especially abundant in amaranth, which helps regulate gastrointestinal function.

It also plays a role in alleviating cold sores. The plant can be applied topically to relieve inflamed skin and lessen swelling.

Amaranth has antioxidant properties due to its high flavonoid content. These have a positive impact on skin health.

Amaranth is rich in the essential amino acid lysine which plays a part in the synthesis of collagen, the absorption of calcium, and the transformation of fat into energy.

Amaranth's application as herbal medicine is due to its high amounts of vitamins and minerals. It is a powerful weight loss herb due to its high protein content and low caloric value, and it also prevents atherosclerosis by preventing an excessive build-up of bad cholesterol (LDL) in the blood vessels. Amaranth has an abundant store of manganese, a mineral that is essential for the metabolism of carbohydrates, encourages calcium absorption, and aids in blood sugar regulation. Amaranth is also a good source of copper, a trace mineral important for body processes such as energy production, brain development, and the maintenance of a healthy white blood cell count.

Amaranth possesses anti-diarrhoeal, astringent, and anti-haemorrhagic actions.

For general health and immunity, an infusion is made with 1 tablespoon of freshly chopped leaves and 1 cup of boiling water. It is steeped for 3 to 5 minutes. This herbal tea is administered in 2 cups daily. This tea is also used as a wash for skin rashes and also gargled for sore mouth and throat.

EUCALYPTUS

Eucalyptus are species of plants that are native to Australia and have also been farmed on plantations throughout many other nations because of their quick growth and they provide valuable timber, pulpwood, honey, and essential oils. The main eucalyptus species used medicinally is the globulus species (commonly known as blue gum), though there are other varieties as well.

The oil extract from the eucalyptus tree is used as antibiotics, perfume, flavouring in cosmetic products, an industrial solvent, and as an ingredient in dental preparations. The oil, which is a colourless liquid with a potent, sweet, woody scent, is extracted from steam distillation of the leaves and branch top. It has eucalyptol, also known as 1,8- cineole.

Eucalyptus has been used for thousands of years in Indian Ayurvedic, Chinese, Greek, and other European medical systems to cure a variety of ailments. The leaves contain flavonoids and tannins, which are plant-based antioxidant and anti-inflammatory agents respectively.

Eucalyptus also contains pinene, cuminaldehyde, and aromadendrene as active constituents.

Mode of Eucalyptus Administration

Eucalyptus is administered topically or via aromatherapy in form of essential oil, tincture, infusion, and ointment. It may also be taken in form of capsules to ease cough and sore throat. Eucalyptus oil may be found in mouthwash, cough syrups, liniments, cough drops, and vaporizer fluids. The leaves are available in three different forms: fresh, dried, and liquid extracts.

Do NOT use orally because it is very poisonous when ingested.

Effects and Uses of Eucalyptus

Eucalyptus is a common ingredient in many medications used to lessen congestion, cold and cough symptoms. Fresh leaves can be gargled with to treat sinusitis, bronchitis, and sore throat. Additionally, it appears that inhaling eucalyptus oil vapour has a decongestant effect. It might work as an expectorant to break up mucus or phlegm and relieve congestion.

It is also present in lotions and ointments used to treat joint and muscle pain. Its pain relief ability is brought about by its flavonoid content which gives it an anti-inflammatory effect.

Eucalyptus has antimicrobial properties due to the presence of cineole which acts as antiseptics and also destroys oral bacteria that can cause bad breath. It has been used in mouthwash and dental treatments because of its antibacterial and antimicrobial properties. It has been used in traditional Aboriginal medicine to treat skin wounds and fungal infections. Eucalyptus oil was employed in hospitals in 19th-century England to clean urinary catheters. Later research confirmed the British use of eucalyptus oil as a cleaning agent by showing that it contains compounds with antimicrobial and antiseptic properties.

Eucalyptus works well both as an insecticide and insect repellent. Some experts recommend using the oil of lemon eucalyptus as an insect repellent since it works well to keep mosquitoes away.

Precautions and Side Effects of Eucalyptus

As long as the oil is diluted, eucalyptus products can be applied to the skin without causing harm. It must first be diluted with a carrier oil, like olive oil, before being applied directly to the skin. One to five drops of essential oil should be used per ounce of carrier oil, or between 1% and 5% of the total mixture should be eucalyptus oil to 95-99% carrier oil.

Both discomfort and a burning sensation can be brought on by eucalyptus. Avoid using it too close to the eyes.

Eucalyptus is very allergic; thus, it is important to get tested before using it. A drop of eucalyptus oil mixed with the carrier oil can be applied to the arm to conduct an allergy test. It is safe to use if there is no reaction after 24 hours. Over time, allergies can arise. Stop using eucalyptus oil if you have used it in the past and now appear to be reacting allergic to it.

Eucalyptus oil is toxic; thus, it cannot be consumed orally.

Diarrhoea, nausea, vomiting, and stomach discomfort are possible side effects of eucalyptus application. Small pupils, breathlessness, and dizziness are symptoms of eucalyptus poisoning. It is crucial to remember that eucalyptus might affect the liver and may combine with other drugs.

Eucalyptus should be used with caution around children because they are more sensitive to essential oils than adults are. Usage should be avoided for pregnant and breastfeeding women.

BEE POLLEN

Bee pollen, also referred to as bee bread and ambrosia, is a ball or pellet of flower pollen that has been collected in the field and packed by worker honeybees. It is a combination of flower pollen, nectar, enzymes, honey, wax, and bee secretions. Simple carbohydrates, protein, minerals, vitamins, fatty acids, and a negligible amount of other compounds make up its composition.

For thousands of years, bee pollen has been utilized medicinally in China. Records of its use date back to 2500 years ago in ancient Greece; Hippocrates, who is frequently referred to as the "father of modern medicine", recommended bee pollen grains for healing. Herbalists have promoted bee pollen as a remedy for a number of illnesses. Due to its excellent nutritional value and abundance of bioactive compounds with antioxidant, anti-inflammatory, and antimicrobial effects, bee pollen is gaining commercial attention. Micronutrients and phenolic compounds are abundant in bee pollen.

Forms of Bee Pollen Administration

Bee pollen can be used as dietary supplements. Bee pollen is ingested by mechanical chewing. It can also be ground into small pieces or heated in warm water to boost its digestibility. It swells in the presence of water, cracks after 2-3 hours, and releases its content Juices from fruits, vegetables, and milk can also be utilized for this. Honey, butter, cottage, cheese, yoghurt, jams, glucose, and other ingredients can be combined with ground pollen in a variety of products at a ratio ranging from 1:1 to 1:4. One teaspoon of mixed pollen is taken three times each day. Enzymatic pollen, however, is advised for usage in several disorders.

Dried pollen can also be taken in form of capsules and extracts. Bee pollen extracts have found topical applications in cosmetics and skin care products.

Effects and Uses of Bee Pollen

Bee pollen is employed in apitherapeutic treatment because it has a range of beneficial effects including antifungal, antibacterial, antiviral, anti-inflammatory, hepatoprotective, immuno-stimulating, and pain relief. It also speeds up the granulation process of wound healing and prevents wound infections.

A range of antioxidants, including flavonoids, carotenoids, kaempferol, quercetin, and glutathione, are abundant in bee pollen. These compounds may shield your cells from the harm done by free radicals, which are connected to a number of chronic diseases, including cancer and type 2 diabetes. Heart disease risk factors like bad LDL cholesterol and lipid oxidation may be reduced by bee pollen.

According to German natural scientist Francis Huber, bee pollen is "the best bodybuilder on earth" since it improves athletic performance. As a result, it is employed by bodybuilders and athletes to boost strength and endurance. It contains all 22 amino acids, which contributes to its reputation as a muscle builder. About half of the amino acids are free-form, which allows for immediate assimilation into the body for use.

Side Effects of Bee Pollen

Consuming bee pollen may come with dangers from pesticides, harmful metals, or fungal mycotoxins contamination. Bee pollen is safe for short-term use; however, allergic reactions could happen in people who have pollen allergies. Allergic reactions include shortness of breath, swelling, hives, and anaphylaxis.

It is not advisable to use bee pollen while nursing or while pregnant. Some bee pollen products have been discouraged from being used by the Food and Drug Administration because they contain unapproved medicines like phenolphthalein and sibutramine.

Bee pollen may also interact with prescriptions and over-the-counter blood-thinning thinning medications such as warfarin (Coumadin). This increases its effects of which are increased chances of bruising and bleeding and a slower time for the blood to clot.

BEESWAX

Beeswax (Cera alba) is made from the honeycomb of the honeybee and other bees. Similar to honey, beeswax has a range of colours based on the bees themselves as well as the flowers that the honey is made from. It comes in three basic varieties: Yellow, White, and Absolute. Their benefits, purposes, and methods of processing all differ. Yellow beeswax is the pure, natural, and unprocessed wax that is extracted from the honeycomb. It goes through filtration, purification, and bleaching process to produce white beeswax. White beeswax is employed in food preparation, pharmaceutical products like ointments and soft-gel capsules, as well as cosmetic formulations and the coating of medication tablets. Yellow beeswax is transformed into Beeswax Absolute by treatment with alcohol.

Forms of Beeswax Administration

Beeswax has topical applications and is also used in aromatherapy. Beeswax is only used externally.

Effects and Uses of Beeswax

Beeswax is a popular ingredient in aromatherapy because of its long, clean, smokeless burn. Along with producing flames that are noticeably brighter, it also helps the removal of airborne impurities and advances both physical and mental well-being in addition to emitting the perfume of honey. It promotes physical and mental well-being by giving the body more energy, lowering stress, improving focus, assisting in the relief of physical discomfort, and controlling blood pressure.

When used topically, beeswax moisturizes, conditions, calms, and soothes the skin. It exfoliates, heals wounds, encourages skin regeneration, lessens the appearance of aging indications, calms itching and irritation, and fortifies a moisturizing, long-lasting barrier of defence against outside pollutants. When applied to hair, beeswax softens, conditions, and nourishes the strands while enhancing their sheen.

When used medicinally, beeswax promotes healing and soothes abrasions. It has anti-inflammatory, anti-allergenic, antibacterial, antiviral, and antioxidant properties. It shields the skin from irritation from the environment and stops hazardous microorganisms from entering the body through chapped or cracked skin.

Precautions and Side Effects of Beeswax

It is advisable to perfume a skin test before using beeswax. Applying melted beeswax the size of a dime to a small, innocuous region of skin and letting it sit there for 15 to 20 minutes will do this. Never put beeswax on skin that is very sensitive, such as the ears, inner nose, or eyes.

Redness, soreness, itching, burning contact dermatitis, shortness of breath, swelling/crusting/rash around the mouth/lips/tongue, small pimples, and difficulties in speaking or swallowing are a few potential adverse effects of beeswax. Avoid using beeswax if you have hay fever, rhinitis, or allergies to pollen, propolis, or honey.

GINKGO BILOBA

Ginkgo biloba, often known as maidenhair, has been utilized in traditional Chinese medicine dating back more than 2000 years ago. Traditional remedies for ginkgo seeds, leaves, and nuts include the treatment of asthma, dementia, bronchitis, kidney, and bladder problems.

Phenolic acids, proanthocyanidins, flavonoid glycosides like myricetin, kaempferol, isorhamnetin, and quercetin, as well as terpene trilactones ginkgolides and bilobalides are all present in ginkgo leaf extracts. Unique ginkgo biflavones, alkylphenols, and polyprenols are also present in the leaves.

Forms of Ginkgo biloba Administration

Ginkgo biloba is administered in the form of capsules, tablets, and liquid extracts. The dried leaves can be used in preparing herbal tea infusions. Raw ginkgo seeds are poisonous and should not be eaten.

Effects and Uses of Ginkgo biloba

Ginkgo biloba displays antihypertensive effect. Ginkgo biloba extract has been proven to lower diastolic blood pressure in hypertensive people when combined with grape seed skin extracts, green tea, quercetin, resveratrol, and bilberry extracts.

The antioxidant property of G. biloba leaf extract makes it one of the most widely used traditional medicinal plants in the treatment of neurological and cardiovascular diseases.

G. biloba seeds are frequently used in traditional Chinese medicine as supplements to treat skin conditions, gonorrhoea, toothaches, and overactive bladders as well as to avoid fever, coughing, and sputum formation.

Ginkgo biloba has anti-inflammatory effects which is beneficial in preventing stroke, arthritis, cancer and heart disease.

By encouraging blood artery dilation, ginkgo biloba can boost blood flow. For the treatment of diseases linked to impaired blood circulation, this may be useful. Ginkgo may be an effective treatment for some headache types due to its capacity to boost blood flow and lessen inflammation.

Ginkgo used orally daily may marginally lessen dementia symptoms and diseases that affect the mind, such as Alzheimer's disease.

Administering Gingko biloba by intravenous medications (IV) in addition to usual therapy can help patients with abrupt hearing loss to hear better. It is unclear whether oral ginkgo is beneficial. Only medical professionals are authorised to administer IV products.

For 8 to 16 weeks, using ginkgo leaf extract orally every day in addition to conventional antipsychotic drugs can alleviate some symptoms of schizophrenia. Additionally, it might lessen antipsychotic medication adverse effects which include thirst, constipation, and the movement disorder – tardive dyskinesia.

Ginkgo extract used orally or intravenously in conjunction with normal therapy appears to enhance thinking, memory, and the capacity to carry out activities of daily living in stroke survivors. Ginkgo extract used orally may not be as effective as one given intravenously. But only a healthcare professional can administer IV products.

Side Effects of Ginkgo biloba

Ginkgo is often safe for healthy individuals to consume in moderation for up to six months. Rarely are there serious negative effects. It may result in a few minor adverse effects, including nausea, headaches, dizziness, and allergic skin reaction. Ginkgo should not be taken if you have an allergy to alkylphenol-containing plants or are on any blood-thinning or antidepressant medications.

When consumed orally, fresh ginkgo seeds and fruits are harmful, fatal, and poisonous. Roasted seeds or crude ginkgo plants on the other hand are edible, but are unsafe and unhealthy when eaten in high quantities and can cause severe negative effects like convulsion.

Ginkgo interacts with prescriptions and over-the-counter medications such as talinolol, efavirenz, alprazolam, ibuprofen, anti-diabetic, anticonvulsant, antidepressant, and anticoagulant drugs. If you take ginkgo together with blood pressure drugs, your blood pressure could fall too low.

Children, pregnant, and breastfeeding women should not take ginkgo.

It should not also be taken by those who have epilepsy as it may result

in seizures.

LEMON

Lemon (Citrus limon) is common for its edible fruit and essential oils. Ascorbic acid (vitamin C), citric acid, d-limonene, and 8-geranyloxypsolaren are key constituents of lemon. Each portion of the plant from which lemon essential oil can be extracted has a different terpene profile. Essential oils can be extracted from the lemon peel of which the limonene and beta-pinene content is usually quite high. Lemon petitgrain oil, which often has higher levels of neral and geraniol, is made from lemon leaves. Lemon blossoms are also sources of essential oils. The limonene content of lemon blossoms was similarly found to be high, but they also contained terpenes including beta-farnesene, alpha-terpinene, alpha-citral, and (E)-ocimene that were not present in the fruit peels or leaves. Of the three sources of lemon essential oil, lemon peel essential oil is the most popular, and it is utilized in aromatherapy for its uplifting and stimulating properties.

Forms of Lemon Administration

Lemon can be administered in the form of hot water extracts (tisane and decoction), cold infusions, liquid extracts, foods (fresh or juiced), capsules, and syrups. Chewing lemon leaves is a traditional remedy for vomiting relief, bile flow stimulation, and cough reduction.

Effects and Uses of Lemon

Numerous phytochemicals, such as polyphenols, terpenes, and tannins are present in lemon. To reduce fever and soothe a sore throat, add lemon and honey to hot water. Lemons contain a lot of d-limonene, which has been demonstrated to be good for the digestive system.

Lemon has antibacterial and immunostimulating actions. Its vitamin C content is helpful in the treatment of scurvy and the prevention of cold and flu. People with anaemia may benefit from the improved iron absorption that lemon can facilitate. Vitamin C enhances the absorption of iron. Lemon's antibacterial property is essential in reducing oral bacteria and canker sores. This makes it frequently found in mouthwash. The antioxidants present in lemon boost the immune system and encourage the development of white blood cells, which can aid in the battle against infections.

Lemon has long been used to stimulate appetite and liver function, as well as to enhance digestion and treat migraine, nausea, and diarrhoea.

Lemon is used in traditional aromatherapy for the relief of stress and fatigue. Citric acid, found in lemons, is a crucial element in the metabolism of fuel. It contributes to the conversion of carbohydrates into cellular energy. This aids in lowering fatigue and stress levels.

Lemon's effectiveness in treating cold and cough symptoms as well as preventing the oral bacteria that causes dental caries and gum disease is largely due to the presence of antibacterial compounds in the oil from lemon peel, such as 8-geranyloxypsolaren.

Because of its high limonene content, lemon has an alkaline effect when eaten orally. This makes it effective for treating inflammatory disorders like arthritis where an excess of acidity is a contributory factor.

Lemon and other citrus fruits contain limonene, which has been used in clinical settings to dissolve cholesterol-containing gallstones. It functions as a natural cholesterol solvent. It has also been used to treat heartburn and gastroesophageal reflux disease (GERD) due to its ability to neutralize gastric acid and encourage proper peristalsis.

Precautions and Side Effects of Lemon

Other than the reactions caused by citrus allergies, lemon has no significant adverse effects. However, in these circumstances, consuming lemons can be extremely risky as repeated consumption may result in a potentially fatal anaphylactic shock.

The use of lemon essential oils is not recommended during pregnancy or lactation.

LAVENDER

Over the years, lavender (Lavandula augustifolia) has been utilized in cosmetics and traditional medicine. The plant is primarily farmed to make lavender essential oil commercially. The essential oil is extracted by distilling the flower spikes. The oil can be used in topical applications, balms, salves, fragrances, and cosmetics. The lavender plant is edible but its essential oil is toxic when taken orally.

Traditional treatments for certain nerve-related diseases, such as insomnia, include lavender preparations. The primary function of lavender flower teas, baths, and pillows in European systems of traditional herbal medicine is as a mild sedative. The lavender preparations are also utilized for their spasmolytic, stomachic, carminative, and diuretic properties in European folk medicine.

The active constituents of lavender are camphor, cinnamaldehyde, linalool, linalyl acetate, borneol, fenchone, geraniol, limonene, linalyl butyrate, tannin, pinene, and cineole. They all work together to deliver the advantages or benefits of lavender. Camphor is responsible for the antiseptic or antimicrobial properties of lavender, whilst cineol has been proven to have analgesic and muscle-relaxing activities. On the other hand, the analgesic, sedative, and anti-inflammatory effects of lavender essential oil when applied topically or inhaled are explained by borneol's interaction with gamma-aminobutyric acid (GABA), a neurotransmitter that regulates fear and anxiety responses as well as the influence of linalool and linalyl acetate over the nervous system.

Forms of Lavender Administration

Lavender can be administered orally in form of dried flowers, herbal tea, tinctures, and capsules. It is used in herbal baths, has topical applications (essential oil, creams, lotions, and poultice), and also in aromatherapy.

Effects and Uses of Lavender

The antiseptic, antifungal, and anti-inflammatory properties of lavender oil can aid in the healing of wounds, minor burns, and insect bites, and in fighting fungal infections such as ringworm and athlete's foot.

Lavender oil might be helpful for treating anxiety, restlessness, depression and sleeplessness. According to scientific research, lavender has mild sedative properties, and lavender aromatherapy may help people with sleep disorders relax, sleep better, and have better moods. It may also slow down nervous system activity. Studies have also shown that massages with lavender oil can help with anxiety reduction, mood stabilization, and better sleep. For the treatment of depression, headaches, and insomnia, add 2-4 drops of lavender oil in 2-3 cups of boiling water then inhale the vapours.

Taking lavender in the form of tea can relieve digestive problems such as nausea, intestinal gas, upset stomach, and abdominal puffiness. It is also used to ease pain from headaches, sprains, toothaches, and sores in addition to aiding with digestive issues. Because lavender oil contains linalyl acetate and linalool (two anti-inflammatory compounds present in many essential oils), it can act as a pain reliever. It can also be applied to tackle hair loss.

Precautions and Side Effects of Lavender

Lavender is safe to use on the skin, however, there is a chance of an allergic reaction or skin irritation as some persons get contact dermatitis, allergic eczema, or face dermatitis. Bumpy skin, redness, or a burning sensation are symptoms of an allergic reaction. If you have sensitivity or reaction, stop usage. When taken orally, lavender may cause headaches, constipation, and changes in appetite. Lavender inhalation may also result in headache, nausea, and chills.

According to the National Institutes of Health (NIH), lavender should not be used with pharmaceuticals that cause drowsiness (such as barbiturates, benzodiazepines, and Ambien) or lower blood pressure (like captopril, enalapril, and losartan). The active constituents of lavender may intensify the effects of sedative and painkiller drugs on the central nervous system.

Additionally, there have been cases where regular use of lavender resulted in prepubertal gynecomastia, a rare disorder that causes increased breast tissue in boys before puberty.

Never apply lavender on an open wound. Get medical help right away. Consult your doctor before using essential oil inhalations (aromatherapy) to determine whether they are appropriate for you if you have asthma. Some people find that using essential oils as inhalants irritates their eyes and/or lungs. Pregnant women and nursing mothers should avoid using lavender.

TEA TREE

The tea tree (Melaleuca alternifolia) is renowned for its essential oil which has both antifungal and antibiotic properties while being safe to use topically. This is commercially produced and marketed as tea tree oil. Tea tree oil, also referred to as Melaleuca oil, is an essential oil with a fresh camphoraceous scent. Its colour can range from pale yellow to almost colourless and transparent. The leaves of the tea tree are the source of its essential oil. The aboriginal people of Australia have long utilized tea tree oil as a herbal remedy and antiseptic. Today, the external application of tea tree oil is encouraged for several ailments including insect bites, athlete's foot, lice, nail fungus, wounds, and acne.

Forms of Tea Tree Administration

Tea tree can be administered both topically (tea tree essential oil and ointments) and via aromatherapy.

Effects and Uses of Tea Tree

Tea tree has anti-inflammatory, antiviral, antifungal, and antibacterial characteristics. Terpinen-4-ol, one of its active constituents, is responsible for these properties. Terpinen-4-ol also boosts the activity of your white blood cells, which aid in fighting infections, wound healing, and warding off pathogens and other foreign invaders.

Tea tree oil can be used to treat head lice, athlete's foot, contact dermatitis, and acne.

Precautions and Side Effects of Tea Tree

Tea tree oil should never be ingested. Oral consumption can cause stomach pain, nausea, vomiting, diarrhoea, extreme rashes, irregular blood cell behaviour, coma, drowsiness, hallucinations, and confusion.

When using tea tree oil on the skin, people must use caution. Application in high doses can irritate the skin or cause contact dermatitis. When using tea tree oil topically, it must always be diluted first in a carrier oil.

intensify the effects of caffeine, which could result in nervousness, sweating, sleeplessness, or irregular heartbeat.

Children, pregnant women, and nursing mothers should not take ginseng.

CLOVES

Cloves (Syzygium aromaticum) have long been used in cooking and traditional medicine. People produce medicine from numerous parts of the clove plant, including the dried buds, stems, and leaves.

In both traditional Chinese and Ayurvedic medicine, cloves have been used to boost the immune system, lessen inflammation, and improve digestion. Clove oil is of high benefit in traditional medicine. Clove oil has long been used to treat respiratory ailments, soothe gastrointestinal discomfort, and relieve pain. Clove oil contains eugenol, a natural antioxidant that reduces oxidative stress, has an anaesthetic effect, and is essential for pain relief. Eugenol has a strong fragrance and gives clove its distinctive scent.

Forms of Clove Administration

Clove is administered topically in form of massage oils, poultices, herbal baths, creams, lotions, or scrubs. It can also be used orally in fresh/whole or dried/ground form and tisanes.

Effects and Uses of Cloves

Clove is classified as an herb. It has many uses and applications in herbalism. To manufacture herbal medicine, people utilize dried flower buds, stems, leaves, and oils. Eugenol in clove oil gives it its antioxidant, analgesic, anaesthetic, and anti-cancer effects. Due to their capacity to reduce oxidative stress, cloves' high antioxidant content may also help prevent liver damage and reduce the risk of diabetes, heart disease, and certain types of cancer. However, eugenol is poisonous in large doses and may harm the liver of children.

The antibacterial properties of cloves may aid in improving oral and dental health. This makes cloves a regular ingredient in toothpaste and mouthwash formulations.

Clove is utilized as an expectorant and for the treatment of stomach upset. Phlegm is easier to cough out when using clove and other expectorants. Bad breath, hernia, and diarrhoea are all treated with clove oil. Cloves also have carminative properties that help to lessen bloating, flatulence, and the excess acidity that can cause heartburn. Clove and its oil are used for treating gastrointestinal gas, nausea, and vomiting. The active ingredients in cloves encourage the formation and secretion of digestive enzymes, which helps with nutrient absorption. Your stomach can be protected from ulcers by using cloves. The thinning of mucus layers lining the stomach can lead to ulcers. Cloves can thicken this mucus, according to preliminary studies, which lowers the chance of getting ulcers and speeds up the healing of existing ones.

For toothaches, to manage pain during dental work, and to treat dry sockets (a complication of tooth extraction), clove is applied topically directly to gums. Additionally, it is used as a counterirritant on the skin to treat discomfort and inflammation in the mouth and throat.

Clove is also administered as a component of a multi-ingredient herbal preparation used to prevent males from premature ejaculation. According to studies, applying a herbal mixture that contains clove flower together with Panax ginseng root, Angelica root, Asiasari root, Torlidis seed, Cistanches deserticola, Zanthoxyl species, cinnamon bark, and toad venom on the skin of the penis greatly improves early ejaculation.

Clove oil may be useful for healing wounds and relieving itching when applied topically. Numerous compounds found in cloves have been associated with anti-inflammatory activities. The most significant of these compounds is eugenol. Eugenol aids in reducing the body's inflammatory response, lowering the likelihood of conditions like arthritis and assisting in the management of symptoms.

Precautions and Side Effects of Cloves

If consumed orally by those who have liver disease, immune system abnormalities, blood clotting disorder, or food allergies, it may have negative effects. Additionally, mouth sensitivity, irritation, and dental tissue damage can be initiated by dry clove.

When applied to the skin, clove oil or cream containing clove flower may be safe. However, using clove oil frequently and repeatedly on the mouth or the gums might occasionally harm the skin, mucous membranes, tooth pulp, and gums.

It is unlikely safe to inhale the smoke from clove cigarettes or administer clove oil intravenously because it can have negative side effects on the lungs like pneumonia and breathing difficulties.

Children should not use herbal remedies containing clove orally as it might cause adverse effects such as fluid imbalance, seizures, and liver damage. If you have peptic ulcer or a bleeding disorder like hemophilia, stay away from clove oil.

The eugenol component of clove oil may slow down the rate at which blood coagulate and clot. Therefore, combining clove oil with anticoagulant, antiplatelet, or blood-thinning medications can have adverse effects such as making bruising and bleeding easier. Individuals on anti-diabetic medications should avoid the use of cloves.

AGRIMONY

Agrimonia eupatoria is a species of agrimony popularly known as common agrimony. The medicinal herb agrimony has a long history of therapeutic applications. It still holds high regard in herbalism as a beneficial plant with various therapeutic uses. Its active constituents are mucilage, bitters, phytosterols and tannins (gallotannins), ursolic acid, palmitic acid, salicylic acid, stearic acid, silicic acid, flavonoids, and tannins. Agrimony has been used for centuries to cure conditions like catarrh, hemorrhage, tuberculosis, and skin conditions. It has reportedly been used in traditional medicine to treat gallbladder issues. In addition, it has been used as dyes, flavouring, anticancer, astringent, cardiotonic, coagulant, diuretic, sedative, and anti-asthmatic agent, as well as to cure corns and warts.

The plant is frequently used in "liver and bile teas" phytomedicine concoctions. In tiny proportions, agrimony extracts are frequently utilized in commercially available European cholagogues, stomach/bowel, and urological medicines.

Forms of Agrimony Administration

Agrimony is administered in the form of tinctures, infusions, liquid extracts, and topicals (essential oil and poultice).

Effects and Uses of Agrimony

Agrimony is categorized as a bitter herb; bitters encourage the creation of stomach acid and enzymes, preparing the digestive tract for the possible assimilation of nutrients from food digested. Agrimony's bitter principles have been used to treat liver cirrhosis and gallstones in Germany. They can also regulate the function of the liver and gallbladder. To support and safeguard the liver, agrimony can be taken as a tonic.

Agrimony's strong tannin content (responsible for its astringent properties) and anti-inflammatory properties make it particularly helpful for the treatment of rashes, burns, hemorrhoids, and a variety of gastrointestinal ailments (notably mild bouts of diarrhoea). Agrimony also referred to as the "gunshot plant", has been used to quicken wound healing and stop bleeding since the Medieval era. This is because of its astringent property. It was used to treat battlefield wounds because it works well as a coagulant, that is, it causes blood to clot. Agrimony is beneficial for lowering body bleeding, including excessive menstrual bleeding, due to this action. Its anti-inflammatory qualities can aid in easing menstruation discomfort brought on by prolonged or heavy bleeding.

Agrimony has a lot of healthy phytochemicals that help the body detoxify. These include tannins, flavan-3-ols, flavonols, flavones, and phenolic acids, all of which have potent antioxidant properties that are beneficial to health. These compounds have been shown to have analgesic and anti-inflammatory properties. Furthermore, the diuretic qualities of agrimony help the kidneys continuously wash out toxins while increasing urine production. This stimulates the kidneys and aids in flushing out uric acid and extra crystals that can accumulate in the body and lead to a variety of issues, including gout, arthritis, and kidney stones.

Agrimony has been used for a very long time to treat upper respiratory tract issues. It is particularly helpful when used as a gargle to treat mouth cancer, swollen gums, and sore throats.

Precautions and Side Effects of Agrimony

Despite being harmless when taken in therapeutic doses, agrimony may cause allergic responses in persons who are sensitive to pollen, such as skin rashes, itching, sneezing, congestion, and exhaustion. Because of its possible effects on the menstrual cycle, agrimony can be unsafe to use during pregnancy.

Agrimony might lower blood sugar levels and may therefore interact with anti-diabetic medications and reduce blood sugar to dangerously low levels. It is suggested to avoid direct sunlight when using agrimony in therapeutic doses because the herb may cause skin sensitivity.

9 798377 190417